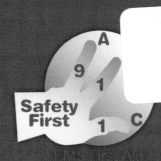

Safety First

# **CPR** Essentials

JONES AND BARTLETT PUBLISHERS

*Sudbury, Massachusetts*

BOSTON   TORONTO   LONDON   SINGAPORE

# Jones and Bartlett Publishers

**World Headquarters**
40 Tall Pine Drive
Sudbury, MA 01776
info@jbpub.com
www.jbpub.com

Jones and Bartlett Publishers Canada
6339 Ormindale Way
Mississauga, Ontario L5V 1J2
Canada

Jones and Bartlett Publishers International
Barb House, Barb Mews
London W6 7PA
United Kingdom

## Toronto EMS
4330 Dufferin Street
Toronto, Ontario M3H 5R9
(416) 392-2000
www.city.toronto.ca/ems

Jones and Bartlett's books and products are available through most bookstores and online booksellers. To contact Jones and Bartlett Publishers directly, call 800-832-0034, fax 978-443-8000, or visit our website www.jbpub.com.

Substantial discounts on bulk quantities of Jones and Bartlett's publications are available to corporations, professional associations, and other qualified organizations. For details and specific discount information, contact the special sales department at Jones and Bartlett via the above contact information or send an email to specialsales@jbpub.com.

**Production Credits**
Chief Executive Officer: Clayton E. Jones
Chief Operating Officer: Donald W. Jones, Jr.
President, Higher Education and Professional Publishing:
  Robert W. Holland, Jr.
V.P., Sales and Marketing: William J. Kane
V.P., Production and Design: Anne Spencer
V.P., Manufacturing and Inventory Control: Therese Connell
Publisher, Public Safety Group: Kimberly Brophy
Acquisitions Editor: Christine Emerton

Reprints Coordinator/Production Assistant: Amy Browning
Photo Research Manager/Photographer: Kimberly Potvin
Director of Sales and Marketing, Canada: Robert Rosenitsch
Interior Design: Anne Spencer
Cover Design: Kristin E. Ohlin
Composition: John Garland
Text Printing and Binding: Courier Kendallville
Cover Printing: Courier Kendallville
Cover Photographs: (left) © Keith Srakocic/AP Photos; (middle) Courtesy of Larry Newell; (right) Courtesy of Larry Newell

The CPR and AED procedures in this book are based on the most current recommendations of responsible medical sources. Toronto EMS and the Publisher, however, make no guarantee as to, and assume no responsibility for, the correctness, sufficiency, or completeness of such information or recommendations. Other or additional safety measures may be required under particular circumstances.

**Library of Congress Catologing-in-Publication Data**
CPR essentials.
    p. cm.
  Includes index.
  ISBN-13: 978-0-7637-5165-4
  ISBN-10: 0-7637-5165-0
  1.  CPR (First aid)--Popular works.
  RC87.9.C748 2007
  616.1'025--dc22
6048                        2007012740

Additional photographic and illustration credits appear on page 51, which constitutes a continuation of the copyright page.
Printed in the United States of America
11  10  09  08  07    10  9  8  7  6  5  4  3  2  1

# Table of Contents

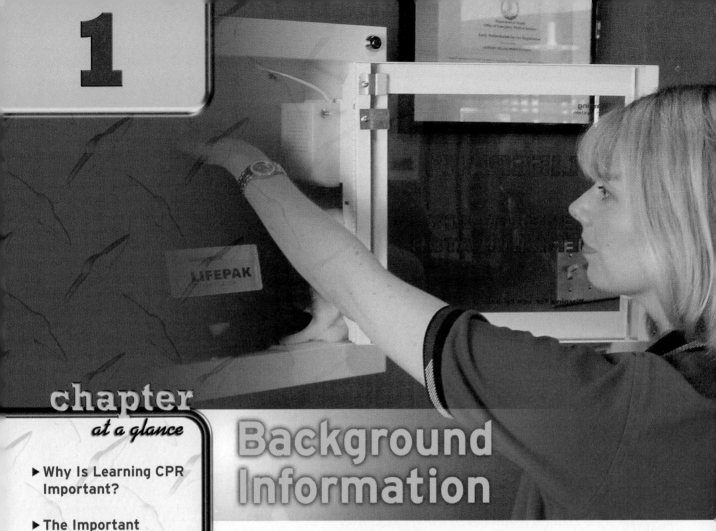

# Background Information

## Why Is Learning CPR Important?

It's better to know CPR and the skill of using an automated external defibrillator and not use it than to need it and not know how to perform it. Everyone should be able to perform CPR and know the basics of using an AED, because when a family member, friend, colleague, or stranger collapses with a cardiac arrest, you may be able to save a life.

A delay of just a few minutes when a person's heart stops can mean the difference between life and death. During their entire lifetimes, most people will see only one or two situations involving life-threatening conditions, but knowing what to do can make a world of difference to the potential survivor.

## The Important Elements of Saving a Life

### Cathy's Story

Cathy, a woman in her mid-forties, was scheduled to attend a conference on May 12, 2005 ( ▶Figure 1-1 ). Her intent was to drive 82 miles to Toronto the night before the conference, spend the night in a hotel, and attend the conference the next day. The day she was to leave, Cathy began to feel unwell. She couldn't put her finger on what was wrong, but did not really feel up to driving to Toronto or attending the conference. Cathy called the hotel to cancel her reservation, but the hotel advised her that the cut-off for canceling reservations had been a half-hour earlier. Cathy did not want to waste the money her employer had spent on the conference and the hotel room, so she decided that she would go to Toronto after all.

Cathy drove, spent the night at the hotel, and got up early the next morning to head over to the conference. She arrived at the conference room a little early and was feeling really poorly. Her jaw was aching and she felt nauseated. Cathy did what everyone does when feeling ill in public; she headed to the washroom for privacy. She sat down in the washroom and put her head in her hands. This was the last thing Cathy remembered until she became aware again several days later in the hospital.

Minutes after Cathy collapsed, some latecomers to the conference stopped in to use the facilities. One of them noticed Cathy and another pressed a panic button in the washroom. The staff were prepared for this moment and immediately responded with an automated external defibrillator in hand.

Cathy was assessed, found to be unresponsive, and not breathing. At the same time, a call was being made to 9-1-1 by the security desk. One of the responders immediately began CPR while the second responder turned on the AED and applied the pads. The AED began analyzing, and within 90 seconds the responders had delivered their first and only shock. Cathy had been in an abnormal heart rhythm called ventricular fibrillation.

Cathy regained signs of life within a minute of receiving CPR and the AED shock. Toronto EMS paramedics arrived and provided advanced care for Cathy during transport to a downtown hospital. Ninety minutes later, Cathy was out of surgery with a stent in place to keep her coronary artery open. Cathy woke up a couple of days later with no recall of the event. The last thing Cathy remembered was feeling unwell in the washroom. She recalls, "When I woke up after the event and someone later handed me my purse, the first thing I noticed was a parking stub for the hotel. I was terrified to think that not only did I have a heart attack, but when we went to Toronto that day, I was driving!" Cathy had no inkling that she had a cardiac problem prior to her sudden cardiac arrest.

Today, this survivor is a vibrant woman with a good job, wonderful children, and many interest and hobbies. She has a lot to live for and a lot of living still to do. Cathy was in the right place at the right time when her sudden cardiac arrest occurred, because the responder at the site had been trained in CPR and AED use and

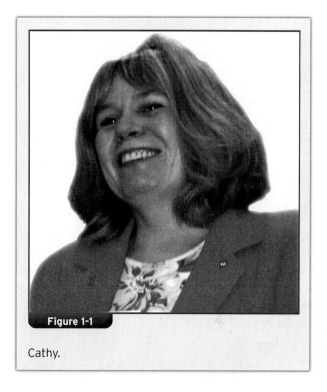

Figure 1-1

Cathy.

had a good emergency response plan in place.

There are many stories similar to Cathy's story. Putting a face to a survivor can really drive home the benefit of knowing CPR and how to use an AED. Every life saved is priceless.

## The Elements of Cathy's Story

Early recognition on the part of the bystanders and the following important elements existed the day Cathy was saved:

1. *Early Access*: The internal emergency response and 9-1-1 were called immediately.

2. *Early CPR*: CPR was initiated immediately.

3. *Early Defibrillation*: An AED was brought to Cathy's side in less than 3 minutes and she was shocked out of the abnormal rhythm and back into an effective normal rhythm.

4. *Early Advanced Care*: Paramedics arrived and began advanced care procedures while en route to the hospital where Cathy was immediately taken into surgery.

These elements are important because they are the basis of emergency cardiac care. Each link in this Chain of Survival is as important as the next. Anyone learning CPR and AED use can increase the chance of survival for victims of sudden cardiac arrest.

# First Aid, CPR, and the Law

Fear of lawsuits has made some people hesitant of becoming involved in emergency situations. First aiders, however, are rarely sued. Following are the legal principles that govern first aid.

## Good Samaritan Laws

In most emergencies, you are not legally required to give first aid. To encourage people to assist others needing help, <u>Good Samaritan laws</u> provide protection against lawsuits. Although laws vary from state to state, Good Samaritan protection generally applies only when the rescuer is:

- Acting during an emergency
- Acting in good faith, which means he or she has good intentions
- Acting without compensation
- Not guilty of malicious misconduct or gross negligence toward the victim (intentionally deviating from established medical guidelines)

Good Samaritan laws are not a substitute for competent first aid or for staying within the scope of your training. To find out about your state's Good Samaritan laws, ask for information at your local library or ask an attorney.

## Duty to Act

<u>Duty to act</u> requires an individual to provide first aid. No one is required to give first aid when no legal duty exists. Duty to act may apply in the following situations:

- *When employment requires it.* If your employer designates you as responsible for providing first aid to meet Occupational Safety and Health Administration (OSHA) requirements and you are called to an emergency, you are required to provide first aid. Examples of occupations that involve a duty to act include law enforcement officers, park rangers, athletic trainers, lifeguards, and teachers ( ▶Figure 1-2 ).

- *When a preexisting responsibility exists.* You may have a preexisting relationship with other persons that makes you responsible for them, which means you must give first aid if they need it. For example, a parent has a preexisting responsibility for a child, and a driver for a passenger.

## Consent

A first aider must have the <u>consent</u> (permission) of a responsive (alert) person before providing care. The victim may give this permission verbally or with a nod of the head (<u>expressed consent</u>). Tell the victim your name, that you have first aid training, and what you would like to do to help.

When the victim is unresponsive (motionless), an adult who is mentally incompetent, or a child with a life-threatening condition whose parent or legal

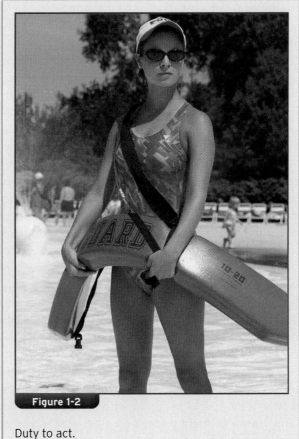

**Figure 1-2**

Duty to act.

guardian is not available, first aiders should assume that <u>implied consent</u> is given. This assumes that the victim (or parent/guardian) would want care provided.

## Abandonment

Once you have started first aid, do not leave the victim until another trained person takes over. Leaving the victim without help is known as <u>abandonment</u>.

## Negligence

<u>Negligence</u> occurs when a victim suffers further injury or harm because the care that was given did not meet the standards expected from a person with similar training in a similar situation. Negligence involves the following:

- Having a duty to act, but either not doing so or doing so incorrectly
- Causing injury and damages

# prep kit

## ▶ Key Terms

**abandonment** Failure to continue first aid until relieved by someone with the same or higher level of training.

**consent** Permission from a victim to allow the first aider to provide care.

**duty to act** An individual's legal responsibility to provide victim care.

**expressed consent** Consent explicitly given by a victim that permits the first aider to provide care.

**Good Samaritan laws** Laws that encourage individuals to voluntarily help an injured or suddenly ill person by minimizing the liability for errors made while rendering emergency care in good faith.

**implied consent** Consent assumed because the victim is unresponsive, mentally incompetent, or underage and has no parent or guardian present.

**negligence** Deviation from the accepted standard of care resulting in further injury to the victim.

## ▶ Assessment in Action

You are driving slowly looking for a house number in an unfamiliar residential area. You are attempting to deliver an important package to a customer. You see an elderly woman lying motionless at the bottom of porch stairs outside a house. You see no one else in the neighborhood, and you are alone. You quickly, but safely, stop your vehicle in front of the victim's house. As you approach the victim, you notice that her skin appears bluish.

*Directions:* Circle Yes if you agree with the statement, and circle No if you disagree.

Yes  No  1. Do you have to stop to help her?

Yes  No  2. You have implied consent to help this person.

Yes  No  3. If she does not respond to your tapping on her shoulders and shouting "Are you OK?" you can leave her and assume that someone else who is more competent or is a family member will arrive shortly to help her.

Yes  No  4. You decide to help. Without examining the victim you quickly straighten her legs, which suddenly causes a bone to protrude through the skin. Would this increase the likelihood of being sued?

*Answers:* 1. No; 2. Yes; 3. No; 4. Yes

## ▶ Check Your Knowledge

*Directions:* Circle Yes if you agree with the statement, and circle No if you disagree.

Yes  No  1. Because an ambulance can arrive within minutes in most locations, most people do not need to learn first aid.

Yes  No  2. Correct first aid can mean the difference between life and death.

Yes  No  3. During your lifetime, you are likely to encounter many life-threatening emergencies.

Yes  No  4. All injured victims need medical care.

Yes  No  5. Before giving first aid, you must get consent (permission) from an alert, competent adult victim.

Yes  No  6. If you ask an injured adult if you can help, and she says "No," you can ignore her and proceed to provide care.

Yes  No  7. People who are designated as first aiders by their employer must give first aid to injured employees while on the job.

Yes  No  8. First aiders who help injured victims are rarely sued.

Yes  No  9. Good Samaritan laws provide a degree of protection for first aiders who act in good faith and without compensation.

Yes  No  10. You are required to provide first aid to any injured or suddenly ill person you encounter.

*Answers:* 1. No; 2. Yes; 3. No; 4. No; 5. Yes; 6. No; 7. Yes; 8. Yes; 9. Yes; 10. No

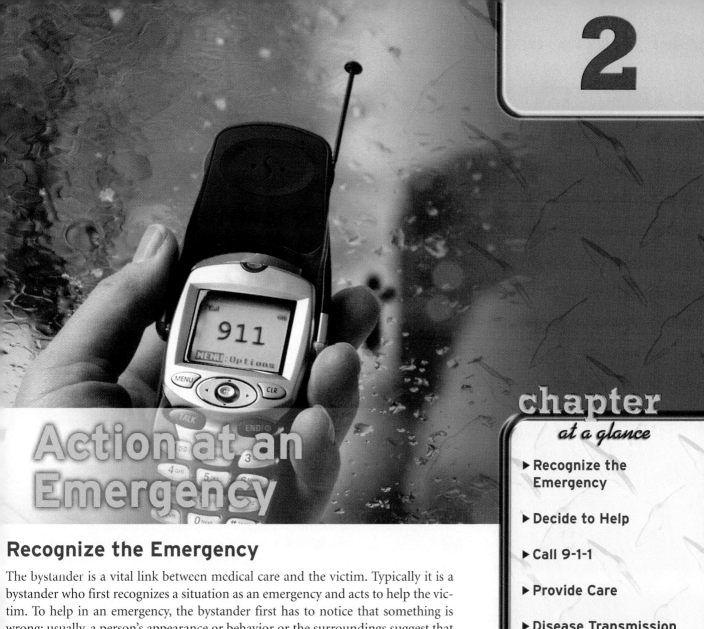

# Action at an Emergency

## Recognize the Emergency

The bystander is a vital link between medical care and the victim. Typically it is a bystander who first recognizes a situation as an emergency and acts to help the victim. To help in an emergency, the bystander first has to notice that something is wrong; usually, a person's appearance or behavior or the surroundings suggest that something unusual has happened.

## Decide to Help

At some point, everyone will have to decide whether to help another person. You will be more likely to get involved if you have previously considered the possibility of helping others. Thus, the most important time to make the decision to help is before you ever encounter an emergency.

### Size Up the Scene

If you are at the scene of an emergency, take a few seconds to briefly survey the scene, considering three things:

1. *Hazards that could be dangerous to you, the victim(s), or bystanders.* Before ap-

## Table 2-1: When to Call 9-1-1

If the answer to any of the following questions is yes, or if you are unsure, call 9-1-1 or your local emergency number for help.

- Is the victim's condition life threatening?
- Could the condition get worse and become life threatening on the way to the hospital?
- Does the victim need the skills or equipment of emergency medical technicians or paramedics?
- Would distance or traffic conditions cause a delay in getting to the hospital?

The following are specific serious conditions for which 9-1-1 should also be called:

- Fainting
- Chest or abdominal pain or pressure
- Sudden dizziness, weakness, or change in vision
- Difficulty breathing or shortness of breath
- Severe or persistent vomiting
- Sudden, severe pain anywhere in the body
- Suicidal or homicidal feelings
- Bleeding that does not stop after 10 to 15 minutes of pressure
- A gaping wound with edges that do not come together
- Problems with movement or sensation following an injury
- Cuts on the hand or face
- Puncture wounds
- The possibility that foreign bodies such as glass or metal have entered a wound
- Most animal bites and all human bites
- Hallucinations and clouding of thoughts
- A stiff neck in association with a fever or a headache
- A bulging or abnormally depressed fontanel (soft spot) in infants
- Stupor or dazed behavior accompanying a high fever
- Unequal pupil size, loss of consciousness, blindness, staggering, or repeated vomiting after a head injury
- Spinal injuries
- Severe burns
- Poisoning
- Drug overdose

*Source:* American College of Emergency Physicians.

proaching the victim(s), scan the area for immediate dangers (such as oncoming traffic, electrical wires, or an assailant). Always ask yourself: Is the scene safe?

2. *Impression of what happened.* Is it an injury or illness, and is it severe or minor?

3. *How many people are involved.* There may be more than one victim, so look around and ask about others who might have been involved.

# Call 9-1-1

Laypersons sometimes make wrong decisions about calling 9-1-1. They may delay calling 9-1-1 or even bypass emergency medical services (EMS) and transport the seriously ill or injured victim to medical care in a private vehicle when an ambulance would have been better for the victim. Some employment situations require that EMS be called rather than having a layperson transport a patient. Fortunately, most injuries and sudden illnesses you encounter will not need more advanced medical care—only first aid. Nevertheless, you should know when to seek medical care.

## When to Seek Medical Care

To know when to seek medical care, you must know the difference between a minor injury or illness and a life-threatening one. For example, upper abdominal pain could be indigestion, ulcers, or an early sign of a heart attack. Wheezing may be related to a person's asthma, for which the person can use his or her prescribed inhaler for quick relief, or it can be a severe, life-threatening allergic reaction to a bee sting.

Not every cut needs stitches, nor does every burn require medical care. However, it is always best to err on the side of caution. When a serious situation occurs, call 9-1-1 *first.* Do not call your doctor, the hospital, or a friend, relative, or neighbor for help before you call 9-1-1. Calling anyone else first only wastes time. ◄ Table 2-1 provides guidance on when to call 9-1-1.

## How to Call 9-1-1

To receive emergency assistance in most communities, you simply dial 9-1-1. Check to see if this is true in your community. Emergency telephone numbers are usually listed on the inside front cover of telephone directories. Keep these numbers nearby or on every telephone. Dial

"0" (the operator) if you do not know the emergency number. When you call 9-1-1, the dispatcher will request certain information:

1. *The victim's location.* Give the address, names of intersecting roads, and other landmarks. Also, tell the specific location of the victim (for example, "in the basement").

2. *The phone number you are calling from and your name.* This prevents false calls and allows a dispatch center without the enhanced 9-1-1 system to call back if you are disconnected or for additional information if needed.

3. *What happened.* State the nature of the emergency (for example, "A worker fell off a ladder and is not moving").

4. *Number of persons needing help and any special conditions* (for example, "There is a liquid spilling from the truck onto the roadway").

5. *Victim's condition* (for example, "He is bleeding from the head") and any care you have provided (such as pressing on the site of the bleeding).

Do *not* hang up the phone until the dispatcher instructs you to do so. The EMS dispatcher may also tell you what to do until EMS arrives. If you send someone else to call, have the person report back to you so you can be sure the call was made.

# Provide Care

Often the most critical life support measures are effective only if started immediately by the nearest available person. That person usually will be a bystander.

# Disease Transmission

The risk of acquiring an infectious disease while providing first aid is very low. But it can be even lower if you know how to protect yourself against diseases transmitted by blood and air.

## Bloodborne Diseases

Some diseases are carried by an infected person's blood (**bloodborne diseases**). Contact with infected blood may result in infection by one of several viruses, such as the following:

- Hepatitis B virus
- Hepatitis C virus
- Human immunodeficiency virus

**Hepatitis** is a viral infection of the liver. Hepatitis B virus (HBV) and hepatitis C virus (HCV) infections result in long-term liver conditions and can lead to liver cancer. Each is caused by a different virus. A vaccine is available for HBV but not for HCV. Employers are required to provide free vaccinations for employees who may be at risk for HBV (for example, health care providers).

A person infected with **human immunodeficiency virus (HIV)** can infect others, and those infected with HIV almost always develop acquired immunodeficiency syndrome (AIDS), which is a major cause of death worldwide. No vaccine is available to prevent HIV infection. The best defense against AIDS is to avoid becoming infected.

## Airborne Diseases

Diseases transmitted through the air by coughing or sneezing (**airborne diseases**) include **tuberculosis (TB)**. TB has increased in frequency and is receiving much attention. TB, which is caused by a bacteria, usually settles in the lungs and can be fatal. In most cases, a first aider will not know that a victim has TB.

Assume that any person with a cough, especially one who is in a nursing home or a shelter, may have TB. Other symptoms include fatigue, weight loss, chest pain, and coughing up blood. If a surgical mask is available, wear it or wrap a handkerchief over your nose and mouth.

## Protection

In most cases, you can control the risk of exposure to diseases by wearing **personal protective equipment (PPE)** and by following some simple procedures. PPE blocks entry of organisms into the body. The most common type of protection involves wearing medical exam gloves ( ▶ **Figure 2-1** ). All first aid kits should have several pairs of gloves. Because some rescuers have allergic reactions to latex, latex-free gloves (vinyl or nitrile) should be available.

Protective eyewear and a standard surgical mask may be necessary in some emergencies; first aiders ordinarily

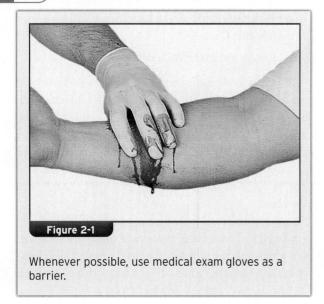

**Figure 2-1**

Whenever possible, use medical exam gloves as a barrier.

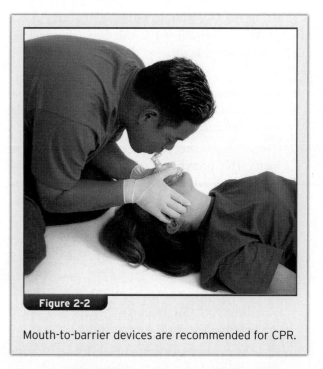

**Figure 2-2**

Mouth-to-barrier devices are recommended for CPR.

will not have or need such equipment. Mouth-to-barrier devices are recommended for cardiopulmonary resuscitation (CPR) ▶Figure 2-2 .

Always assume that *all* blood and body fluids are infected. Protect yourself even if blood or body fluids are not visible. At the workplace, PPE must be accessible, and your employer must provide training to help you choose the right PPE for your work.

First aiders can protect themselves and others against diseases by following these steps:

1. Wear appropriate PPE, such as gloves. If they are not available, put your hands in plastic bags or use waterproof material for protection.

2. If you have been trained in the correct procedures, use absorbent barriers to soak up blood or other infectious materials.

3. Clean the spill area with an appropriate disinfecting solution, such as diluted bleach (one fourth cup of bleach in a gallon of water).

4. Discard contaminated materials in an appropriate waste disposal container.

5. Wash your hands with soap and water after giving first aid.

6. If the exposure happened at work, report the incident to your supervisor. Otherwise, contact your personal physician.

## Rescuer Reactions

After providing care for severe injuries or illnesses, rescuers may feel an emotional letdown. Stressful events can be psychologically overwhelming and may result in a condition known as <u>post-traumatic stress disorder</u>. Its symptoms include depression and flashbacks. Discussing your feelings, fears, and reactions within 24 to 72 hours of helping at a traumatic injury scene helps prevent later emotional problems. You could discuss your feelings with a trusted friend, a mental health professional, or a member of the clergy. Quickly bringing out your feelings helps relieve personal anxieties and stress.

## ▶ Key Terms

**airborne diseases** Infections transmitted through the air, such as tuberculosis.

**bloodborne diseases** Infections transmitted through the blood, such as HIV or hepatitis B virus.

**hepatitis** A viral infection of the liver.

**human immunodeficiency virus (HIV)** The virus that causes acquired immunodeficiency syndrome (AIDS).

**personal protective equipment (PPE)** Equipment, such as medical exam gloves, used to block the entry of an organism into the body.

**post-traumatic stress disorder** A psychological disorder that may occur after a stressful event; symptoms include depression and flashbacks.

**tuberculosis (TB)** A bacterial disease that usually affects the lungs.

## ▶ Assessment in Action

You are rushing parts to one of your largest customer's broken machines. Because time is money, the customer is losing a lot for each hour the machine is down. It's beginning to rain. Suddenly, you see a motorcyclist skid off the highway and into a ditch. You have a cellular telephone in your car.

*Directions*: Circle Yes if you agree with the statement, and circle No if you disagree.

Yes No 1. As you approach the victim, you should not be concerned about any other possible victims.

Yes No 2. This crash scene could be dangerous.

Yes No 3. In most communities, 9-1-1 can be used to contact the EMS.

Yes No 4. Expect to give your name when you call 9-1-1.

Yes No 5. If you do not know the exact address of the emergency, be prepared to give a description of the location as best as you can.

*Answers:* 1. No; 2. Yes; 3. Yes; 4. Yes; 5. Yes

## ▶ Check Your Knowledge

*Directions*: Circle Yes if you agree with the statement, and circle No if you disagree.

Yes No 1. A scene survey should be done before giving first aid to an injured victim.

Yes No 2. For a severely injured victim, call the victim's doctor before calling for an ambulance.

Yes No 3. Dial "0" (for the telephone operator) if you do not know the emergency telephone number.

Yes No 4. First aiders should assume that blood and all body fluids are infectious.

Yes No 5. If you are exposed to blood while on the job, report it to your supervisor, and if off the job, to your personal physician.

Yes No 6. First aid kits should contain medical exam gloves.

Yes No 7. Wash your hands with soap and water after giving first aid.

Yes No 8. Vaccinations are available for both HBV and HCV.

Yes No 9. Medical exam gloves can be made of almost any material as long as they fit the hand well.

Yes No 10. Tuberculosis is a bloodborne disease.

*Answers:* 1. Yes; 2. No; 3. Yes; 4. Yes; 5. Yes; 6. Yes; 7. Yes; 8. No; 9. No; 10. No

# How the Body Functions

## The Respiratory System

The body can store food to last several weeks and water to last several days, but it can store enough oxygen for only a few minutes. Ordinarily this does not matter because we have only to inhale air to get the oxygen we need. If the body's oxygen supply is cut off, as in drowning, choking, or smothering, death will result in about four to six minutes unless the oxygen intake is restored. Oxygen from air is made available to the blood through the <u>respiratory system</u> and then to the body cells by the circulatory system.

### Nose

Air normally enters the body during inhalation through the nostrils. It is warmed, moistened, and filtered as it flows over the damp, sticky lining (mucous membrane) of the nose. When a person breathes through the mouth instead of the nose, there is less filtration and warming. After passing through the nasal passages, air enters the nasal portion of the pharynx (throat).

### Pharynx and Trachea

From the back of the nose or the mouth, the air enters the throat or pharynx

▶Figure 3-1. The pharynx is a common passageway for food and air. At its lower end, the pharynx divides into two passageways, one for food and the other for air. Muscular control in the back of the throat routes food to the food tube (<u>esophagus</u>), which leads to the stomach; air is routed from the pharynx to the windpipe (<u>trachea</u>), which leads to the lungs. The trachea and the esophagus are separated by a small flap of tissue (epiglottis), which diverts food away from the trachea. Usually this diversion works automatically to keep food out of the trachea and to prevent air from entering the esophagus. If the muscles of the pharynx and larynx are not coordinated, food or other liquid can enter the trachea instead of the esophagus.

However, normal swallowing controls do not operate if a person is unconscious. *That is why a first aider should never pour liquid into the mouth of an unconscious person in an attempt to revive him or her. The liquid may flow down into the windpipe and suffocate the victim.* Foreign objects, such as false teeth or a piece of food, may also lodge in the throat or windpipe and cut off the passage of air.

In the upper two inches of the trachea, just below the epiglottis, is the voice box (<u>larynx</u>), which contains the vocal cords. The larynx can be felt in the front of the throat (<u>Adam's apple</u>).

## Lungs

The trachea branches into two main tubes (bronchial tubes or bronchi), one for each lung. Each bronchus divides and subdivides somewhat like the branches of a tree. The smallest bronchi end in thousands of tiny pouches (<u>alveoli</u> or air sacs), just as the twigs of a tree end in leaves. Each air sac is enclosed in a network of capillaries. The walls that separate the air sacs and the capillaries are very thin. Through those walls, oxygen combines with hemoglobin in red blood cells to form oxyhemoglobin, which is carried to all parts of the body. Carbon dioxide and certain other waste gases in the blood move across the capillary walls into the air sacs and are exhaled from the body. The lungs occupy most of the chest cavity.

## Mechanics of Breathing

The passage of air into and out of the lungs is called res-

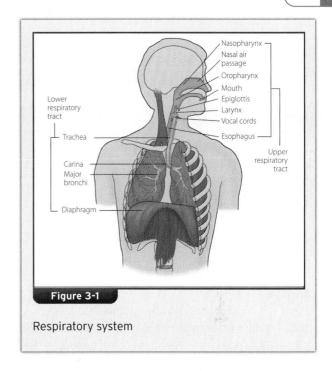

**Figure 3-1**

Respiratory system

piration. Breathing in is called inhalation; breathing out is exhalation.

Respiration is a mechanical process brought about by alternately increasing and decreasing the size of the chest cavity. When the <u>diaphragm</u> (the dome-shaped muscle dividing the chest from the <u>abdomen</u>) contracts, the chest expands, drawing air into the lungs (inhalation). An exchange of oxygen and carbon dioxide takes place in the lungs. When the diaphragm expands, it exerts pressure on the lungs, causing air to flow out (exhalation).

Infants and children differ from adults. Their respiratory structures are smaller and more easily obstructed than those of adults. Infants' and children's tongues take up proportionally more space in the mouth than do adults'. The trachea is more flexible in infants and children. The primary cause of cardiac arrest in infants and children is an uncorrected respiratory problem.

The average rate of breathing in an adult at rest is 12 to 20 complete respirations per minute ▶Table 3-1. Normal rates for children are from 15 to 30 times per minute; infant rates will be between 25 and 50 times per minute. Normally the rate slows when a person is lying down and speeds up during vigorous exercise. The rate

| Table 3-1: Normal Respiration Rate Ranges | |
| --- | --- |
| **Breaths per Minute*** | |
| Adults | 12 to 20 |
| Children | 15 to 30 |
| Infants | 25 to 50 |

*To obtain the breathing rate in a person, count the number of breaths in a 30-second period and multiply by 2. Avoid letting the person know you are counting to prevent influencing the rate.

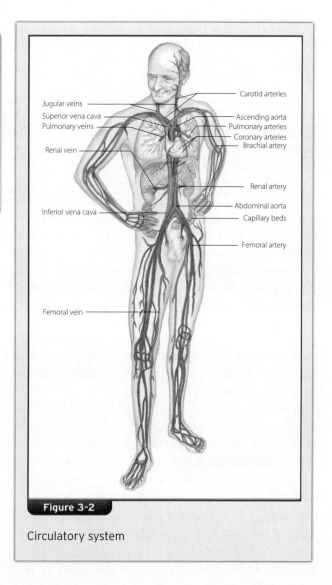

**Figure 3-2**

Circulatory system

of breathing is controlled by a nerve center in the brain (the respiratory center).

Signs of inadequate breathing include a rate of breathing outside normal ranges, cool or clammy skin with a pale or cyanotic (blue-gray) color, and nasal flaring, especially in children.

When a person performs hard muscular work, the lungs cannot get rid of carbon dioxide or take in oxygen fast enough at the normal rate. As carbon dioxide increases in the blood and tissues, the respiratory center sends impulses along its nerves to cause deeper and more rapid respirations. At the same time, the heart rate increases. This increases the supply of oxygen available to the body, as the heart pumps more blood through the lungs.

# The Circulatory System

The circulatory system (▶Figure 3-2) is made up of the blood, the heart, and the blood vessels. Blood is the great delivery system for cells throughout the body. It carries nutrients and other products from the digestive tract in its plasma, and oxygen from the lungs in its hemoglobin. It also transports wastes produced by the cells to the lungs, kidneys, and other excretory organs for removal from the body.

## Heart

The human circulatory system is a completely closed circuit of tubelike vessels through which blood flows. The heart (▶Figure 3-3), by contracting and relaxing,

pumps blood through the vessels. It is a powerful, hollow, muscular organ about as big as a man's clenched fist, shaped like a pear, and located in the left center of the chest, behind the sternum (breast bone). The heart is divided by a wall in the middle. Right and left compartments are divided into two chambers, atrium above, ventricle below. Check valves are located between each atrium and its corresponding ventricle and at the exit of the major arteries leading out of each ventricle. The opening and shutting of these valves at just the right time in the heartbeat keeps the blood from backing up.

At each beat, or contraction, the heart pumps blood

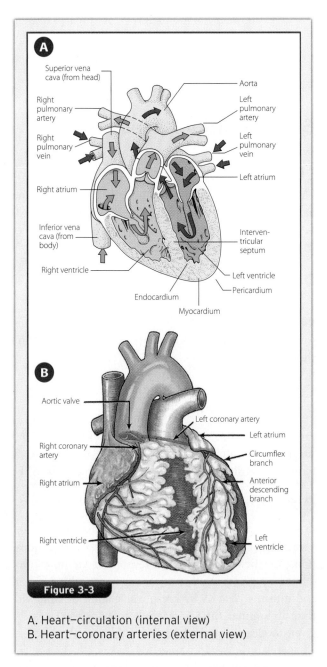

**Figure 3-3**

A. Heart–circulation (internal view)
B. Heart–coronary arteries (external view)

| Table 3-2: Normal Heart Rates | |
| --- | --- |
| Breaths per Minute* | |
| Adults | 60 to 100 |
| Children | 80 to 100 |
| Toddlers | 100 to 120 |
| Newborns | 120 to 140 |

*To obtain a heart rate in most people, count the number of beats over a 30-second period and multiply by 2.

## Blood Vessels

The **arteries** are elastic, muscular tubes that carry blood away from the heart. They begin at the heart as two large tubes: the pulmonary artery, which carries blood to the lungs for the carbon dioxide–oxygen exchange, and the aorta, which carries blood to all the other parts of the body. The **aorta** divides and subdivides until it ends in networks of extremely fine vessels (**capillaries**) smaller than hairs. Through the thin walls of the capillaries, oxygen and food pass out of the bloodstream into the stationary cells of the body, while the body cells discharge their waste products into the bloodstream. In the capillaries of the lungs, carbon dioxide is released and oxygen is absorbed. Capillaries, having reached their limit of subdivision, begin to join together again into **veins**. The veins become larger and larger and finally form major trunks that empty blood returning from the body into the right atrium and blood from the lungs into the left atrium.

It is impossible to prick normal skin anywhere without puncturing capillaries. Because the flow of blood through the capillaries is relatively slow and under little pressure, blood merely oozes from a punctured capillary and usually has time to clot, promptly plugging the leak.

Each time the heart contracts, the surge of blood can be felt as a **pulse** at any point where an artery lies close to the surface of the body, near the skin surface and over a bone. When an artery is cut, blood spurts out. There is no pulse in a vein because the pulse is lost by the time the blood has passed through the capillaries. Hence, blood from a cut vein flows out in a steady stream. It has much less pressure behind it than blood from a cut artery.

rich in carbon dioxide and low in oxygen from the right ventricle to the lungs and returns oxygen-rich blood to the left atrium of the heart. The left ventricle pushes blood rich in oxygen freshly obtained to the rest of the body and returns oxygen-poor blood to the right atrium. At each relaxation of the heart, blood flows into the left atrium from the lungs and into the right atrium from the rest of the body ▶Table 3-2.

# Shock

<u>Shock</u> refers to circulatory system failure, which happens when insufficient amounts of oxygenated blood is provided for every body part. Because every injury affects the circulatory system to some degree, first aiders should automatically treat injured victims for shock.

To understand shock, think of the circulatory system as having three components: a working pump (the heart), a network of pipes (the blood vessels), and an adequate amount of fluid (the blood) pumped through the pipes. Damage to any of these components can deprive tissues of blood and produce the condition known as shock.

Shock can be classified as one of three types according to which component fails.

- *Pump failure*: the heart cannot pump sufficient blood. For example, a major heart attack can damage the heart muscle so the heart cannot squeeze and therefore cannot push blood through the blood vessels.
- *Fluid loss*: a significant amount of fluid, usually blood, is lost from the system.
- *Pipe failure*: blood vessels (pipes) enlarge and the blood supply is insufficient to fill them. This can result when the nervous system is damaged, such as with a spinal injury or drug overdose).

## What to Look For

- altered mental status: anxiety and restlessness
- pale, cold, and clammy skin, lips, and nail beds
- nausea and vomiting
- rapid breathing and pulse
- unresponsiveness when shock is severe

## What to Do

Even if an injured victim does not have signs or symptoms of shock, first aiders should treat for shock.

1. Treat life-threatening injuries and other severe injuries.
2. Lay the victim on his or her back.
3. Raise the victim's legs 8 to 12 inches. Raising the legs allows the blood to drain from the legs back to the heart.
4. Prevent body heat loss by putting blankets and coats under and over the victim ▶Figure 3-4.

# 6-Step Initial Assessment

## Scene Safety

Make sure that the scene is safe and that there are no hazards to you, the victim, or the bystanders. Hazards can include fire, smoke, gas, broken glass, downed electrical wires, and traffic.

## Determine Unresponsiveness

Call the victim in a tone of voice that is loud enough for the victim to hear. If the victim does not respond to the sound of your voice, gently tap or shake the victim's shoulder.

## Call 9-1-1 and Activate Internal Emergency Response System

Ensure that someone has called 9-1-1 and if you are at a site that has internal responders, make sure that they have been notified as well. Have someone bring the AED.

## Open Airway

In an unresponsive victim, the airway must be open for breathing. If the victim is alert and able to answer questions, the airway is open. If a responsive victim cannot talk or cough forcefully, the airway is probably blocked and must be cleared. In a responsive adult or child victim, abdominal thrusts (Heimlich maneuver) can be given to clear a blocked airway. This step is covered in Chapter 4.

In an unresponsive victim lying face up, open the airway using the head tilt-chin lift method. Once the victim's airway is open, the initial check can continue. If the victim is lying face down, carefully turn the victim onto his/her back to complete your assessment.

## Breathing

In this step you check to see if the victim is breathing and, if so, if he or she is having any obvious difficulty

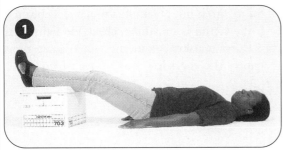

1. Usual shock position. Elevate the legs 8 to 12 inches (if spinal injury is not suspected).

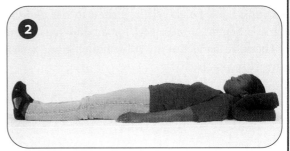

2. Elevate the head for head injury (if spinal injury not suspected).

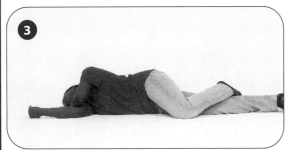

3. Lay an unresponsive, breathing victim on his or her side.

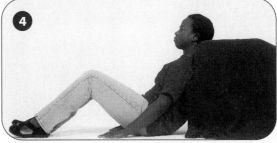

4. Use a half-sitting position for those with breathing difficulties, chest injuries, or a heart attack.

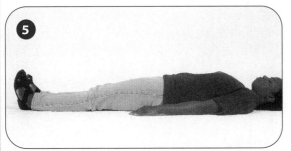

5. Keep victim flat if a spinal injury is suspected or victim has leg fractures.

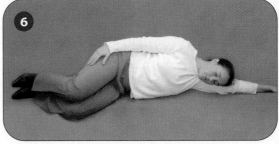

6. Use the high arm in endangered spine (HAINES) position by extending the victim's arm above the head, bending both of the victim's knees, and rolling the victim to their side onto the extended arm.

**Figure 3-4**

Positioning the shock victim

breathing. While holding the airway of the unresponsive victim open, look, listen, and feel for breathing for 5 to 10 seconds. Look for the victim's chest to rise and fall. Listen for breath sounds. Feel for air moving against your cheek. If the victim is not breathing, give 2 rescue breaths (1 second each).

## Circulation

If the victim **is not** breathing immediately begin CPR.

If the victim **is** breathing, check for signs of circulation including skin colour and temperature, movement or pulse. Also check for signs of severe bleeding.

## ▶ Vital Vocabulary

<u>abdomen</u> The body cavity that contains the major organs of digestion and excretion. It is located below the diaphragm and above the pelvis.

<u>Adam's apple</u> The projection on the anterior surface of the neck, formed by the thyroid cartilage over the larynx.

<u>alveoli</u> The air sacs of the lungs in which the exchange of oxygen and carbon dioxide takes place.

<u>aorta</u> The principal artery leaving the left side of the heart and carrying freshly oxygenated blood to the body.

<u>arteries</u> A blood vessel, consisting of three layers of tissue and smooth muscle, that carries blood away from the heart.

<u>capillary</u> The small blood vessels through whose walls various substances pass into and out of the tissues and onto the cells.

<u>circulatory system</u> The arrangement of connected tubes, including the arteries, arterioles, capillaries, venules, and veins, that moves blood, oxygen, nutrients, carbon dioxide, and cellular waste throughout the body.

<u>diaphragm</u> A muscular dome that forms the undersurface of the thorax, separating the chest from the abdominal cavity. Contraction of the diaphragm brings air into the lungs. Relaxation allows air to be expelled from the lungs.

<u>esophagus</u> A collapsible tube that extends from the pharynx to the stomach; contractions of the muscle in the wall of the esophagus propel food and liquids through it to the stomach.

<u>heart</u> A hollow muscular organ that receives blood from the veins and propels it into the arteries.

<u>larynx</u> The voice box.

<u>pulse</u> The wave of pressure created as the heart contracts and forces blood out the left ventricle and into the major arteries.

<u>respiratory system</u> All the structures of the body that contribute to the process of breathing, consisting of the upper and lower airways and their component parts.

<u>shock</u> Inadequate tissue oxygenation resulting from serious injury or illness.

<u>trachea</u> The windpipe; the main trunk for air passing to and from the lungs.

<u>vein</u> Any blood vessel that carries blood from the tissues to the heart.

## ▶ Assessment in Action

Thanks to your friendly and engaging first aid and CPR instructor, you now have a firm grasp on how the human body works. Now you can watch those medical shows and decode some of their dialogue! As you settle into the couch next to your roommate to watch your favorite medical drama, you wonder if you'll ever have another opportunity to apply your new knowledge. During a commercial, such an opportunity arises when your roommate begins making coughing noises and slumps forward.

*Directions:* Circle Yes if you agree with the statement, circle No if you disagree.

Yes   No   **1.** There is no cause to panic; the human body can survive for an hour without oxygen.

Yes   No   **2.** You should pinch your roommate's nose to see if he'll start breathing through his mouth.

Yes   No   **3.** Since your roommate's chest is not moving, he is not breathing.

# prep kit

Yes   No   **4.** If your roommate is not breathing, his body is not getting enough carbon dioxide into the lungs.

*Answers:* **1.** No; **2.** No; **3.** Yes; **4.** No

## ▶ Check Your Knowledge

*Directions:* Circle Yes if you agree with the statement, circle No if you disagree.

Yes   No   **1.** The human body can store oxygen for hours.

Yes   No   **2.** The heart is a pear-shaped, muscular organ.

Yes   No   **3.** Anxiety and restlessness are signs of shock.

*Answers:* **1.** No; **2.** Yes; **3.** No

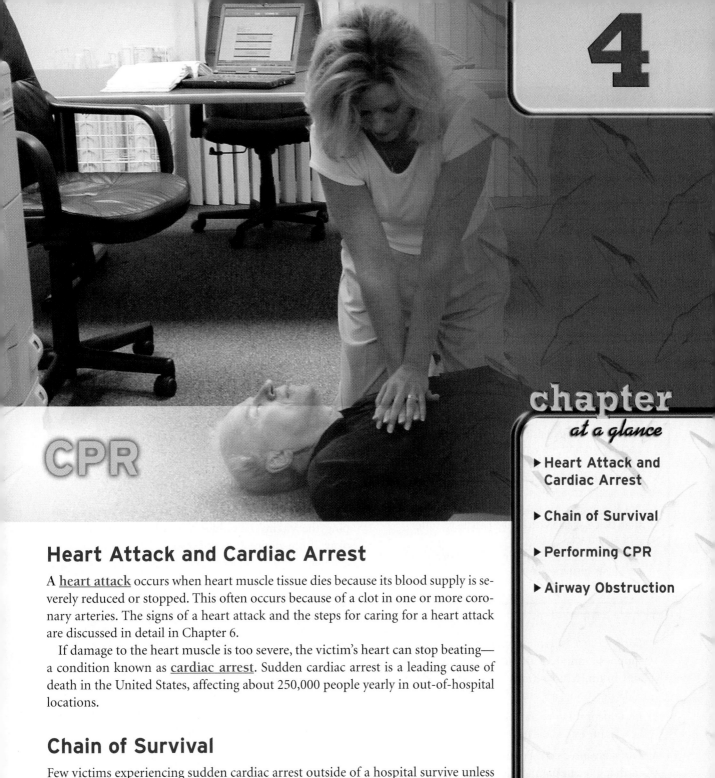

# CPR

## Heart Attack and Cardiac Arrest

A <u>heart attack</u> occurs when heart muscle tissue dies because its blood supply is severely reduced or stopped. This often occurs because of a clot in one or more coronary arteries. The signs of a heart attack and the steps for caring for a heart attack are discussed in detail in Chapter 6.

If damage to the heart muscle is too severe, the victim's heart can stop beating—a condition known as <u>cardiac arrest</u>. Sudden cardiac arrest is a leading cause of death in the United States, affecting about 250,000 people yearly in out-of-hospital locations.

## Chain of Survival

Few victims experiencing sudden cardiac arrest outside of a hospital survive unless a rapid sequence of events takes place. The <u>chain of survival</u> is a way of describing the ideal sequence of care that should take place when a cardiac arrest occurs.

The four links in the chain of survival are as follows:

1. *Early access*: Recognizing early warning signs and immediately calling 9-1-1 to activate emergency medical services (EMS).

## FYI

### Risk Factors of Cardiovascular Disease

Several factors contribute to an increased risk of developing heart disease. Risk factors you cannot change are as follows:

- *Heredity:* Tendencies appear in family lines.
- *Gender:* Men have a greater risk. Even after menopause, when women's death rate from heart disease increases, it is never as high as men's.
- *Age:* Over 80% of those who die from heart disease are 65 or older.

### Risk factors you can change are as follows:

- *Tobacco smoking:* Smokers have a two to four times greater chance of developing heart disease than nonsmokers.
- *High blood pressure:* This condition increases the heart's workload.
- *High cholesterol:* Too much cholesterol can cause a buildup on the walls of the arteries.
- *Diabetes:* This condition affects blood cholesterol and triglyceride levels.
- *Overweight and obesity:* Excess body fat, especially around the waist, increases the likelihood of developing heart disease. Being overweight affects blood pressure and cholesterol and places an added strain on the heart.
- *Physical inactivity:* Inactive people are more than twice as likely as active people to suffer a heart attack.
- *Stress:* Excessive, long-term stress can create problems in some people.

## FYI

### Defibrillation

Most adults in cardiac arrest need defibrillation. Early defibrillation is the single most important factor in surviving cardiac arrest. Chapter 5 provides information on automated external defibrillators (AEDs).

2. *Early CPR*: Cardiopulmonary resuscitation (CPR) supplies a minimal amount of blood to the heart and brain. It buys time until a defibrillator and EMS personnel are available.

3. *Early defibrillation*: Administering a shock to the heart can restore the heartbeat in some victims.

4. *Early advanced care*: Paramedics provide advanced cardiac life support to victims of sudden cardiac arrest. This includes providing IV fluids, medications, and advanced airway devices.

If any one of these links in the chain is broken (absent), the chance that the victim will survive is greatly decreased. If all links in the chain are strong, the victim has the best possible chance of survival.

# Performing CPR

When a person's heart stops beating, he or she needs CPR, an AED, and EMS professionals quickly. CPR consists of breathing oxygen into a victim's lungs and moving blood to the heart and brain by giving **chest compressions**. CPR techniques are very similar for infants (birth to 1 year), children (ages 1–8), and adults (age 8 and older), with just a few slight variations.

## Check for Responsiveness

When the scene is safe, check for responsiveness by tapping the victim's shoulder and asking if he or she is okay. If the victim does not respond, ask a bystander to call 9-1-1. If you are alone with an adult and a phone is nearby, call 9-1-1. If you are alone with an unresponsive child or infant, give CPR for five cycles (2 minutes), then call 9-1-1.

## Open the Airway and Check for Breathing

Place the victim face up on a hard surface. Before starting CPR, open the victim's airway and check for normal breathing. Open the airway by tilting the head back and lifting the chin ▶Figure 4-1 . This moves the tongue away from the back of the throat, allowing air to enter and escape the lungs. The procedure can be done for injured or uninjured victims.

While performing the head tilt–chin lift maneuver, check for breathing by placing your ear next to the victim's mouth. Look at the victim's chest for rise and fall and listen and feel for other signs of normal breathing for 5 to 10 seconds ▶Figure 4-2 .

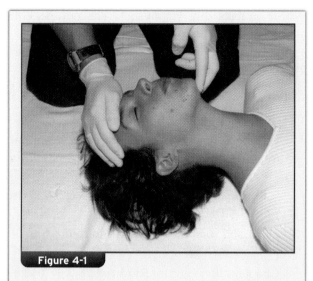

**Figure 4-1**

The head tilt–chin lift maneuver is a simple method for opening the airway.

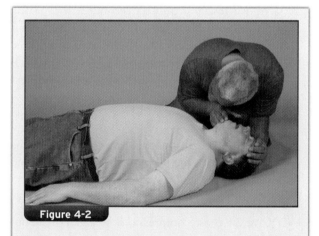

**Figure 4-2**

Look, listen, and feel for signs of normal breathing.

## Rescue Breaths

If the victim is not breathing, you must provide <u>rescue breaths</u>. With the airway open, pinch the victim's nose and make a tight seal over the victim's mouth with your mouth. Give one breath lasting 1 second, take a normal breath for yourself, and then give another breath like the first one. Each rescue breath should make the victim's chest rise. Other methods of rescue breathing are as follows:

- Mouth-to-barrier device
- Mouth-to-nose method
- Mouth-to-stoma method

### Mouth-to-Barrier Device

A barrier device is placed in the victim's mouth or over the victim's mouth and nose as a precaution against infection. There are several different types of barrier devices, and all are easy to use with little modification to the mouth-to-mouth method ▶ Figure 4-3 .

### Mouth-to-Nose Method

If you cannot open the victim's mouth, the victim's mouth is severely injured, or you cannot make a good seal with the victim's mouth (for example, because there are no teeth), use the mouth-to-nose method. With the head tilted back, push up on the victim's chin to close the mouth. Make a seal with your mouth over the victim's nose and provide rescue breaths.

### Mouth-to-Stoma Method

Some diseases of the vocal cords may result in surgical removal of the larynx. People who have this surgery breathe through a small permanent opening in the neck called a stoma. To perform mouth-to-stoma breathing, close the victim's mouth and nose and breathe through the opening in the neck.

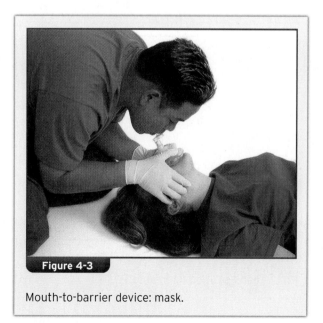

**Figure 4-3**

Mouth-to-barrier device: mask.

## Chest Compressions

Chest compressions move a minimal amount of blood to the heart and brain. Perform chest compressions with two hands for an adult, one or two hands for a child, and two fingers for an infant. Effective compressions require rescuers to push hard and fast. The chest of an adult should be compressed 1.5 to 2 inches, and the chest of a child or infant should be compressed one third to one half the depth of the chest. The desired position for adult and child chest compressions is in the center of the chest between the nipples; for infants, it is just below the nipple line ( ▼ **Figure 4-4** ).

Give 30 compressions at a rate of 100 compressions per minute for adults, children, and infants. After 30 compressions, give two rescue breaths. Repeat the cycles of 30 compressions and two breaths for five total cycles (2 minutes). Continue the cycles of CPR until an AED

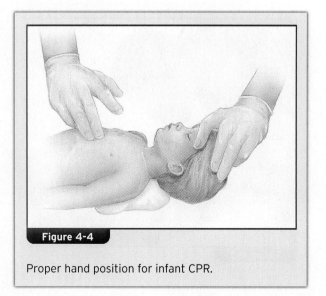

**Figure 4-4**

Proper hand position for infant CPR.

becomes available, the victim shows signs of life, EMS takes over, or you are too tired to continue.

Over the years, CPR procedures have become easier for people to learn and remember.

### Adult CPR

To perform adult CPR, follow these steps ( ▶ **Skill Scan** ):

1. Check responsiveness by tapping the victim and asking, "Are you okay?" If unresponsive, roll the victim onto his or her back.

2. Have someone call 9-1-1 and have someone else retrieve an AED if available.

3. Open the airway using the head tilt–chin lift method (Step **1** ).

4. Check for breathing for 5 to 10 seconds by looking for chest rise and fall and listening and feeling for breathing (Step **2** ). If the victim is breathing, place him or her in the recovery position. If the victim is not breathing, go to the next step.

5. Give two rescue breaths (1 second each), making the chest rise (Step **3** ). If the first breath does not make the chest rise, retilt the head and try the breath again and then proceed to the next step. If both breaths make the chest rise, go to the next step.

6. Perform CPR (Step **4** ).

   • Place the heel of one hand on the center of the chest between the nipples. Place the other hand on top of the first hand.

   • Depress the chest 1.5 to 2 inches.

   • Give 30 chest compressions at a rate of about 100 per minute.

   • Open the airway, and give two breaths (1 second each).

7. Continue cycles of 30 chest compressions and two breaths until an AED is available, the victim starts to move, EMS takes over, or you are too tired to continue.

### Child CPR

To perform CPR on a child, follow these steps ( ▶ **Skill Scan** ):

1. Check responsiveness by tapping the victim and

# Skill Scan

## Adult CPR

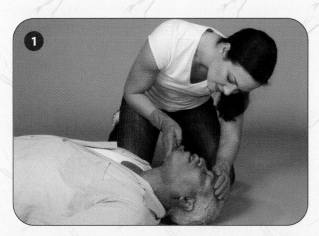

**1.** Open the airway using the head tilt–chin lift method.

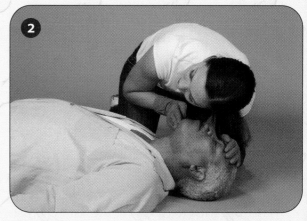

**2.** Check for breathing for 5 to 10 seconds. If the victim is breathing, place him or her in the recovery position. If the victim is not breathing, go to the next step.

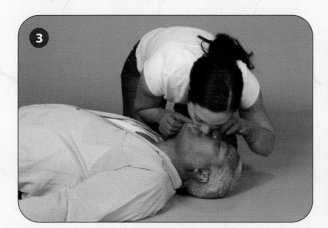

**3.** Give two rescue breaths (1 second each).
If the first breath does not make the chest rise, retilt the head and try the breath again and then proceed to the next step. If both breaths make the chest rise, go to the next step.

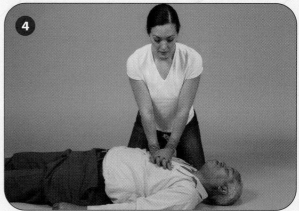

**4.** Perform CPR.

shouting, "Are you okay?" If unresponsive, roll the victim onto his or her back.

2. Have someone call 9-1-1 and have someone else retrieve an AED if available.

3. Open the airway using the head tilt–chin lift method (Step **1**).

4. Check for breathing for 5 to 10 seconds by looking for chest rise and fall and listening and feeling for breathing (Step **2**). If the victim is breathing, place him or her in the recovery position. If the victim is not breathing, go to the next step.

5. Give two rescue breaths (1 second each), making the chest rise (Step **3**). If the first breath does not cause the chest to rise, retilt the head and try the breath again and then proceed to the next step. If both breaths cause the chest to rise, go to the next step.

6. Perform CPR.

   • Place one hand (Step **4**) or two hands on the center of the chest between the nipples. If two hands are used, place one hand on top of the other as in adult CPR.

   • Depress chest one third to one half the depth of the chest.

   • Give 30 chest compressions at a rate of about 100 per minute.

   • Open the airway and give two breaths (1 second each).

7. Continue cycles of 30 chest compressions and two breaths until an AED is available, the victim starts to move, EMS takes over, or you are too tired to continue.

### Infant CPR

To perform CPR on an infant, follow these steps ( ▶ Skill Scan ):

1. Check responsiveness by tapping the victim and shouting, "Are you okay?" If unresponsive, roll the victim onto his or her back.

2. Have someone call 9-1-1.

3. Open the airway by tilting the head back slightly and lifting the chin (Step **1**).

4. Check breathing for 5 to 10 seconds by looking for

chest rise and fall and listening and feeling for breathing (Step **2**). If the victim is breathing, place him or her in the recovery position. If the victim is not breathing, go on to the next step.

5. Give two rescue breaths (1 second each), making the chest rise (Step **3**). If the first breath does not cause the chest to rise, retilt the head and try the breath again and then proceed to the next step. If both breaths cause the chest to rise, go to the next step.

6. Perform CPR (Step **4**).

   • Place two fingers on the breastbone just below the nipple line (one finger even with the line).

   • Depress chest one third to one half the depth of the chest.

   • Give 30 chest compressions at a rate of about 100 per minute.

   • Open the airway and give two breaths (1 second each).

7. Continue cycles of 30 chest compressions and two breaths until the infant starts to move, EMS arrives, or you are too tired to continue.

## FYI

### Compression-Only CPR

Mouth-to-mouth rescue breathing has a long safety record for victims and rescuers. But fear of infectious diseases causes some to be reluctant to give mouth-to-mouth rescue breaths to strangers.

To avoid the chance that the victim will not receive any care, compression-only CPR can be considered in these circumstances:

• Rescuer is unwilling or unable to perform mouth-to-mouth rescue breathing.

• Untrained bystander is following dispatcher-assisted CPR instructions.

## Airway Obstruction

People can choke on all kinds of objects. Foods such as candy, peanuts, and grapes are major offenders because of their shapes and consistencies. Nonfood choking deaths are often caused by balloons, balls and marbles, toys, and coins inhaled by children and infants.

# Skill Scan

## Child CPR

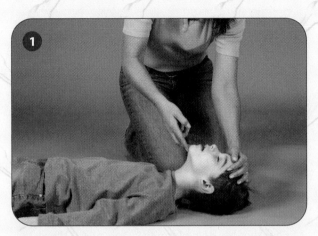

**1.** Open the airway using the head tilt--chin lift method.

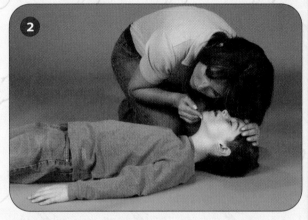

**2.** Check for breathing for 5 to 10 seconds. If the victim is breathing, place him or her in the recovery position. If the victim is not breathing, go to the next step.

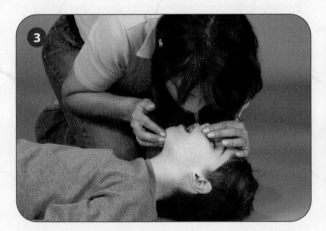

**3.** Give two rescue breaths (1 second each). If the first breath does not make the chest rise, retilt the head and try the breath again and then proceed to the next step. If both breaths make the chest rise, go to the next step.

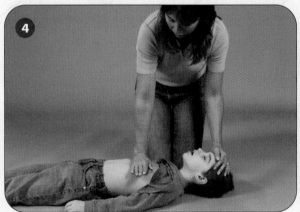

**4.** Perform CPR using either one or two hands.

# Skill Scan

## Infant CPR

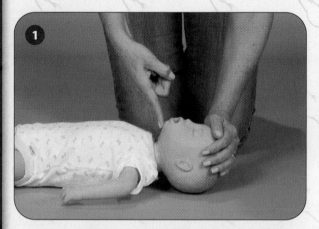

1. Open the airway by tilting the head back slightly and lifting the chin.

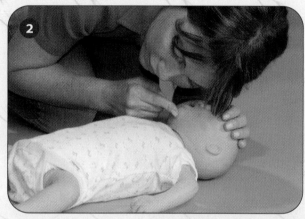

2. Check for breathing for 5 to 10 seconds. If the victim is breathing, place him or her in the recovery position. If the victim is not breathing, go to the next step.

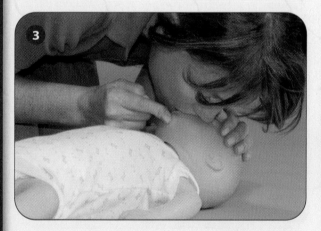

3. Give two rescue breaths (1 second each). If the first breath does not make the chest rise, retilt the head and try the breath again and then proceed to the next step. If both breaths make the chest rise, go to the next step.

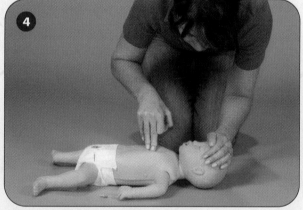

4. Perform CPR.

## Recognizing Airway Obstruction

An object lodged in the airway can cause a mild or severe **airway obstruction**. In a mild airway obstruction, good air exchange is present. The victim is able to make forceful coughing efforts in an attempt to relieve the obstruction. The victim should be encouraged to cough.

A victim with a severe airway obstruction will have poor air exchange. The signs of a severe airway obstruction include the following:

- Breathing becoming more difficult
- Weak and ineffective cough
- Inability to speak or breathe
- Skin, fingernail beds, and the inside of the mouth appear bluish gray (indicating cyanosis)

Choking victims may clutch their necks to communicate that they are choking. This motion is known as the universal distress signal for choking. The victim becomes panicked and desperate ( ▶Figure 4-5 ).

## Caring for Airway Obstruction

For a responsive adult or child with a severe airway obstruction, ask the victim "Are you choking?" If the victim is unable to respond, but nods yes, provide care for the victim. Move behind the victim and reach around the victim's waist with both arms. Place a fist with the

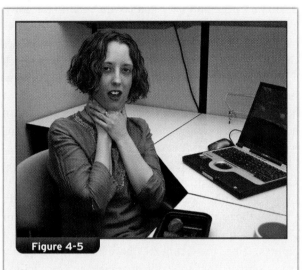

**Figure 4-5**

The universal sign of choking.

thumb side against the victim's abdomen, just above the navel. Grasp the fist with your other hand and press into the abdomen with quick inward and upward thrusts (Heimlich maneuver). Continue thrusts until the object is removed or the victim becomes unresponsive.

For a responsive infant with a severe airway obstruction, give back blows and chest thrusts instead of abdominal thrusts to relieve the obstruction. Support

## CPR

### Unresponsive Victim?

- Open the airway: Head tilt-chin lift.
- Check for breathing: Look, listen, and feel.

**Not Breathing**

- Have someone call 9-1-1 and get an AED if available (for adults and children)
- Give two breaths.
- If first breath does not make chest rise, retilt head and try second breath.
- Whether second breath is successful or not, perform CPR: 30 compressions and two breaths. For airway obstruction, look for object in mouth before giving two breaths and remove if seen.

**Breathing**

- Place victim in recovery position.

the infant's head and neck and lay the infant face down on your forearm, then lower your arm to your leg. Give five back blows between the infant's shoulder blades with the heel of your hand. While supporting the back of the infant's head, roll the infant face up and give five chest thrusts with two fingers on the infant's sternum in the same location used for CPR. Repeat these steps until the object is removed or the infant becomes unresponsive.

If you are caring for an unresponsive, nonbreathing victim of any age and your first breath does not make the chest rise, retilt the head and try a second breath. Whether the second breath is successful or not, perform CPR: 30 compressions and two breaths for five cycles (2 minutes). Since the victim may have had a foreign body airway obstruction, look for an object in the victim's mouth and, if seen, remove it before giving the two breaths during the cycles of CPR.

To relieve airway obstruction in a responsive adult or child who cannot speak, breathe, or cough, follow the steps in ( ►Skill Scan ):

1. Check victim for choking by asking, "Are you choking? (Step ❶).

2. Have someone call 9-1-1.

3. Position yourself behind the victim and locate the victim's navel (Step ❷).

## FYI

### The Tongue and Airway Obstruction
Airway obstruction in an unresponsive victim lying on his or her back is usually the result of the tongue relaxing in the back of the mouth, restricting air movement. Opening the airway with the head tilt–chin lift method may be all that is needed to correct this problem.

4. Place a fist with thumb side against the victim's abdomen just above the navel (Step ❸), grasp it with the other hand, and press into victim's abdomen with quick inward and upward thrusts (Step ❹). Continue thrusts until the object is removed or the victim becomes unresponsive.

If the victim becomes unresponsive, call 9-1-1 and give CPR. Each time you open the airway to give a breath, look for an object in the mouth or throat and, if seen, remove it.

To relieve airway obstruction in a responsive infant who cannot cry, breathe, or cough, follow the steps in ( ►Skill Scan ):

1. Have someone call 9-1-1.

2. Support the infant's head and neck and lay the infant face down on your forearm, then lower your arm to your leg. Give five back blows between the infant's shoulder blades with the heel of your hand (Step ❶).

3. While supporting the back of the infant's head, roll the infant face up and give five chest thrusts on the infant's sternum in same location used in CPR (Step ❷).

4. Repeat these steps until the object is removed. If the infant becomes unresponsive, begin CPR. Each time you open the airway to give a breath, look for an object in the mouth or throat and, if seen, remove it.

# Skill Scan

## Airway Obstruction in a Responsive Adult or Child

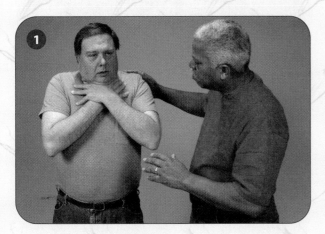

**1.** Check victim for choking.

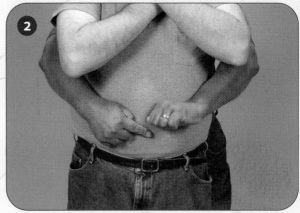

**2.** Locate the navel.

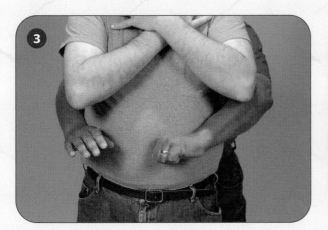

**3.** Place thumb side of fist just above the navel.

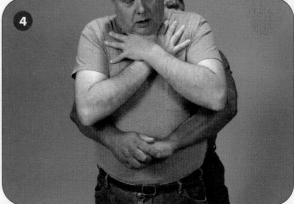

**4.** Place other hand on top of first hand and give abdominal thrusts until object is removed.

# Skill Scan

## Airway Obstruction in a Responsive Infant

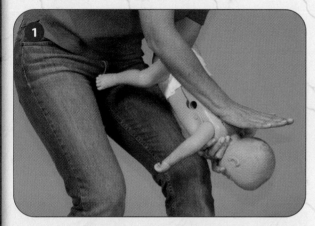

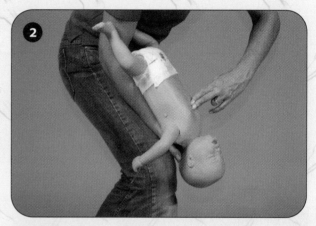

1. Support the infant's head, neck, and back. Give five back blows.

2. Give five chest thrusts.

# CPR and Airway Obstruction Review

**These steps are the same for all victims regardless of age:**

- Check responsiveness: Tap a shoulder and ask if the victim is okay. If unresponsive, have someone call 9-1-1.
- Open airway: Head tilt–chin lift maneuver.
- Check for breathing: Look at the chest to see it rise and fall, and listen and feel for breathing (5–10 seconds).
- If victim is breathing but unresponsive, place him or her in recovery position.
- If victim is not breathing, give two breaths (1 second per breath).
- If breaths make the chest rise, begin CPR: cycles of 30 chest compressions and two breaths for five cycles (2 minutes) at a rate of 100 compressions per minute. Recheck breathing after every five cycles.
- If first breath does not make the chest rise, retilt victim's head and try a second breath.
- If the second breath does not make the chest rise (do not give more than two breaths), assume that the airway is obstructed: Give cycles of 30 chest compressions, look for object in the mouth, remove any visible object, and give two breaths.

| Action | Adult (≥8 years) | Child (1–8 years) | Infant (<1 year) |
|---|---|---|---|
| 1. Breathing methods | Mouth-to-barrier device Mouth-to-mouth Mouth-to-nose Mouth-to-stoma | Mouth-to-barrier device Mouth-to-mouth Mouth-to-nose Mouth-to-stoma | Mouth-to-mouth and nose Mouth-to-barrier device Mouth-to-mouth Mouth-to-nose Mouth-to-stoma |
| 2. Chest compressions | | | |
|    Locations | On the breastbone, between nipples | On the breastbone, between nipples | On the breastbone, just below nipple line |
|    Method | Two hands: Heel of one hand on chest; other hand on top | One or two hands (depending on size of victim and rescuer) | Two fingers |
|    Depth | 1.5 to 2 inches | One third to one half the depth of the chest | One third to one half the depth of the chest |
|    Rate | 100 per minute | 100 per minute | 100 per minute |
|    Ratio of chest compressions to breaths | 30:2 | 30:2 | 30:2 |
| 3. When to activate EMS when alone | Immediately after determining victim is unresponsive. | After performing five cycles (2 minutes) of CPR | After performing five cycles (2 minutes) of CPR |
| 4. Use of AED | Yes; Deliver one shock as soon as possible, followed immediately by 5 cycles of CPR. | Yes; Deliver one shock as soon as possible, followed by 5 cycles of CPR. Use pediatric pads if available. | No |
| 5. Responsive victim and airway obstruction | Abdominal thrusts (Heimlich maneuver) | Abdominal thrusts (Heimlich maneuver) | Alternate five back blows followed by five chest thrusts repeatedly |

# prep kit

## ▶ Key Terms

<u>airway obstruction</u> A blockage, often the result of a foreign body, in which air flow to the lungs is reduced or completely blocked.

<u>cardiac arrest</u> Stoppage of the heartbeat.

<u>chain of survival</u> A four-step concept to help improve survival from cardiac arrest: early access, early CPR, early defibrillation, and early advanced care.

<u>chest compressions</u> Depressing the chest and allowing it to return to its normal position as part of CPR.

<u>CPR</u> Cardiopulmonary resuscitation; the act of providing rescue breaths and chest compressions for a victim in cardiac arrest.

<u>heart attack</u> Death of a part of the heart muscle.

<u>rescue breaths</u> Breathing for a person who is not breathing.

## ▶ Assessment in Action

You are at a local health club when you overhear someone in the weight room nearby shouting for help. You enter the room and see a person lying motionless on the floor. You quickly confirm that he is unresponsive.

*Directions:* Circle Yes if you agree with the statement, and circle No if you disagree.

Yes No 1. The next thing to do is to start chest compressions.

Yes No 2. The ratio of chest compressions to rescue breaths is 15 to 2.

Yes No 3. Compression depth for an adult is one third the depth of the chest.

Yes No 4. Open the airway using the head tilt–chin lift method.

Yes No 5. Continue CPR until an AED becomes available or EMS personnel arrive.

*Answers:* 1. No; 2. No; 3. No; 4. Yes; 5. Yes

## ▶ Check Your Knowledge

*Directions:* Circle Yes if you agree with the statement, and circle No if you disagree.

Yes No 1. Take 5 to 10 seconds when checking for breathing.

Yes No 2. If an adult victim is unresponsive, the next step is to call 9-1-1.

Yes No 3. Tilting the head back and lifting the chin helps move the tongue and open the airway.

Yes No 4. If you determine that a victim is not breathing, begin chest compressions.

Yes No 5. Do not start chest compressions until you have checked for a pulse.

Yes No 6. For all victims (adult, child, infant) needing CPR, give 30 compressions followed by two breaths.

Yes No 7. Use two fingers when performing CPR on an infant.

Yes No 8. A sign of choking is that the victim is unable to speak or cough.

Yes No 9. To give abdominal thrusts to a responsive choking victim, place your fist below the victim's navel.

Yes No 10. When giving abdominal thrusts to a responsive choking victim, repeat the thrusts until the object is removed or the victim becomes unresponsive.

*Answers:* 1. Yes; 2. Yes; 3. Yes; 4. No; 5. No; 6. Yes; 7. Yes; 8. Yes; 9. No; 10. Yes

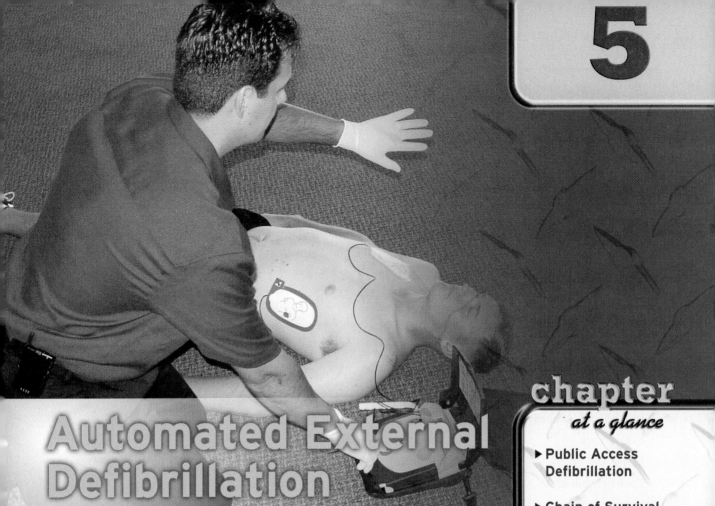

# Automated External Defibrillation

## Public Access Defibrillation

Sudden cardiac death remains an unresolved public health crisis. A victim's chance of survival dramatically improves through early cardiopulmonary resuscitation (CPR) and early <u>defibrillation</u> with the use of an <u>automated external defibrillator (AED)</u>. To be effective, defibrillation must be used in the first few minutes following cardiac arrest. The implementation of state public access defibrillation (PAD) laws and the Food and Drug Administration's (FDA) approval of "home use" AEDs have made this important care step available to many rescuers in many places, including the following ( ▶Figure 5-1 ):

- Airports and airplanes
- Stadiums
- Health clubs
- Golf courses
- Schools
- Government buildings
- Offices
- Homes

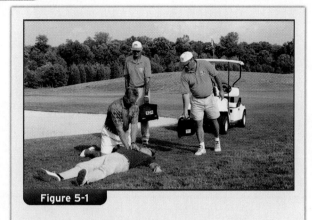

**Figure 5-1**

AEDs are available in many places for use by trained rescuers.

## Chain of Survival

The chain of survival is a concept that recognizes the importance of four critical components in saving the life of a victim of cardiac arrest. Early defibrillation is the third link in this chain ( ▼ Figure 5-2 ):

1. Early access
2. Early CPR
3. Early defibrillation
4. Early advanced care

## How the Heart Works

The heart is an organ with four hollow chambers. The two chambers on the right side receive blood from the body and send it to the lungs for oxygen. The two chambers on the left side of the heart receive freshly oxy-

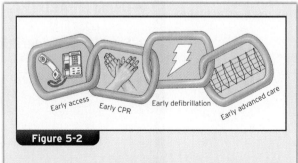

**Figure 5-2**

Defibrillation is a critical link in the chain of survival.
*Source:* American Heart Association.

genated blood from the lungs and send it back out to the body.

The heart has a unique electrical system that controls the rate at which the heart beats and the amount of work the heart performs. In the right upper chamber of the heart, there is a collection of special pacemaker cells. These cells emit electrical impulses about 60 to 100 times a minute that cause the other heart muscle cells to contract in a coordinated manner ( ▼ Figure 5-3 ).

Because the heart contracts approximately every second, it needs an abundant supply of oxygen, which it gets through the coronary arteries. These arteries run along the outside of the heart muscle and branch into smaller vessels. These arteries sometimes become diseased (atherosclerosis), resulting in a lack of oxygen to the pacemaker cells, which can cause abnormal electrical activity in the heart.

## When Normal Electrical Activity Is Interrupted

Ventricular fibrillation (also known as *V-fib*) is the most common abnormal heart rhythm in cases of sudden cardiac arrest in adults ( ►Figure 5-4 ).

The organized wave of electrical impulses that cause the heart muscle to contract and relax in a regular fashion is lost when the heart is in ventricular fibrillation. As

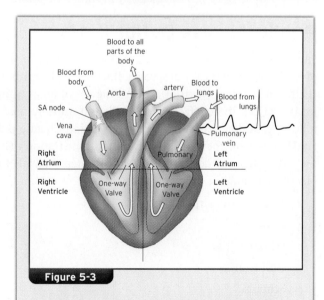

**Figure 5-3**

The sinoatrial (SA) node is the primary heart pacemaker, which sends electrical impulses to contract the heart's chambers in a coordinated manner.

a result, the lower chambers of the heart quiver and cannot pump blood, so circulation is lost (no pulse).

A second, potentially life-threatening, electrical problem is ventricular tachycardia (*V-tach*), in which the heart beats too fast to pump blood effectively ▼ Figure 5-5 .

## Care for Cardiac Arrest

When the heart stops beating, the blood stops circulating, cutting off all oxygen and nourishment to the entire body. In this situation, time is a crucial factor. For every minute that defibrillation is delayed, the victim's chance of survival decreases by 7% to 10% ▶ Figure 5-6 .

CPR is the initial care for cardiac arrest, until a defibrillator is available. Perform cycles of chest compressions and breaths until an AED is ready to be connected to the victim.

## About AEDs

An AED is an electronic device that analyzes the heart rhythm and if necessary delivers an electric shock, known as defibrillation, to the heart of a person in cardiac arrest. The purpose of this shock is to correct one of the abnormal electrical disturbances previously discussed and to reestablish a heart rhythm that will result in normal electrical and pumping function.

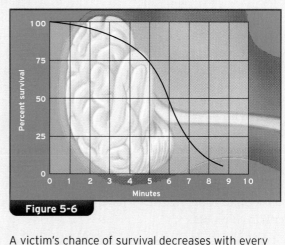

Figure 5-6

A victim's chance of survival decreases with every minute that passes without proper care.

All AEDs are attached to the victim by a cable connected to two adhesive pads (electrodes) placed on the victim's chest. The pad and cable system sends the electrical signal from the heart into the device for analysis and delivers the electric shock to the victim when needed ▼ Figure 5-7 .

AEDs have built-in rhythm analysis systems that determine whether the victim needs a shock. This system

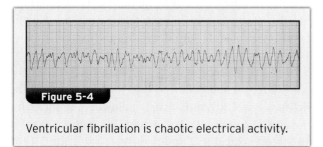

Figure 5-4

Ventricular fibrillation is chaotic electrical activity.

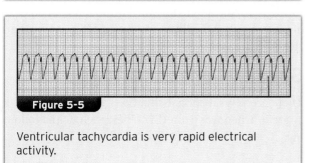

Figure 5-5

Ventricular tachycardia is very rapid electrical activity.

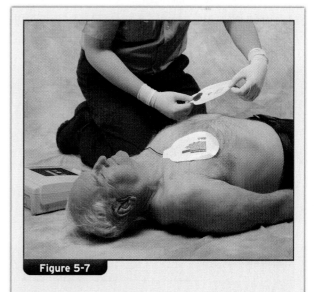

Figure 5-7

Two adhesive pads are placed on the victim's chest and connected by a cable to the AED.

enables first aiders and other rescuers to deliver early defibrillation with only minimal training.

AEDs also record the victim's heart rhythm (known as an electrocardiogram, or ECG), shock data, and other information about the device's performance (for example, the date, time, and number of shocks supplied) **▼ Figure 5-8** .

## Common Elements of AEDs

Many different AED models exist. The principles for use are the same for each, but the displays, controls, and options vary slightly. You will need to know how to use your specific AED. All AEDs have the following elements in common:

- Power on/off mechanism
- Cable and pads (electrodes)
- Analysis capability
- Defibrillation capability
- Prompts to guide you
- Battery operation for portability

# Using an AED

Once you have determined the need for the AED (victim unresponsive and not breathing), the basic operation of all AED models for anyone over 1 year of age follows this sequence **▶Skill Scan** :

1. Perform CPR until an AED is available (Step **1** ).

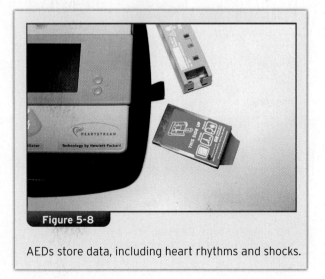

**Figure 5-8**

AEDs store data, including heart rhythms and shocks.

2. Once the AED is available, turn the equipment on.
3. Apply the electrode pads to the victim's bare chest and the cable to the AED (Step **2** ). Use child pads for a child if available.
4. Stand clear and analyze the heart rhythm.
5. Deliver a shock if indicated (Step **3** ).
6. Perform CPR for five cycles (2 minutes).
7. Check the victim and repeat the analysis, shock, and CPR steps as needed (Step **4** ).

Some AEDs power on by pressing an on/off button. Others power on when opening the AED case lid. Once the power is on, the AED will quickly go through some internal checks and will then begin to provide voice and screen prompts.

Expose the victim's chest. The skin must be fairly dry so that the pads will adhere and conduct electricity properly. If necessary, dry the skin with a towel. Because excessive chest hair may also interfere with adhesion and electrical conduction, you may need to quickly shave the area where the pads are to be placed.

Remove the backing from the pads and apply them firmly to the victim's bare chest according to the diagram on the pads. One pad is placed to the right of the breastbone, just below the collarbone and above the right nipple. The second pad is placed on the left side of the chest, left of the nipple and above the lower rib margin.

Make sure the cable is attached to the AED, and stand clear for analysis of the heart's electrical activity. No one should be in contact with the victim at this time, or later if a shock is indicated.

The AED will advise if a shock is needed. Deliver the shock after verifying that no one is in contact with the victim. Begin CPR immediately following the shock for five cycles (2 minutes). Following CPR, recheck to see if the victim is breathing and reanalyze the rhythm. If the shock worked, the victim will begin to regain signs of life. Continue providing care until EMS personnel arrive and take over.

# Special Considerations

There are several special situations that you should be aware of when using an AED. These include the following:

- Water

# Skill Scan

## Using an AED

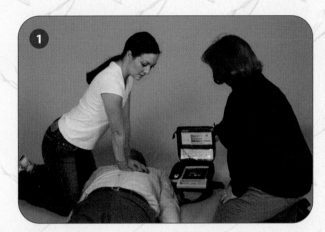

1. Perform CPR until AED is available.

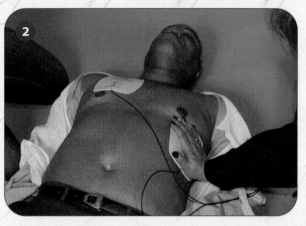

2. Turn on the device and attach AED pads and cable.

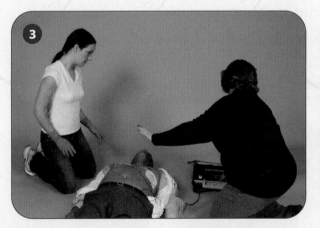

3. Stand clear and analyze rhythm. Shock if advised.

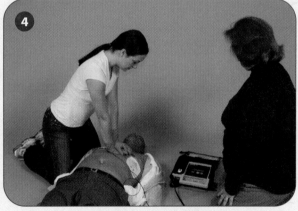

4. Perform CPR for five cycles (2 minutes) and recheck victim.

- Children
- Medication patches
- Implanted devices

## Water

Because water conducts electricity, it may provide an energy pathway between the AED and the rescuer or bystanders. Remove the victim from free-standing water. Quickly dry the chest before applying the pads. The risk to the rescuers and bystanders is very low if the chest is dry and the pads are secured to the chest.

## Children

Cardiac arrest in children is usually caused by an airway or breathing problem, rather than a primary heart problem as in adults. AEDs can deliver energy levels appropriate for children aged 1 year or older. If your AED has special pediatric pads and cable, use these for the child ( ▼ Figure 5-9 ). If the pediatric equipment is not available, use the adult equipment.

## Medication Patches

Some people wear an adhesive patch containing medication (such as nitroglycerin, nicotine, or pain medication) that is absorbed through the skin. Because these

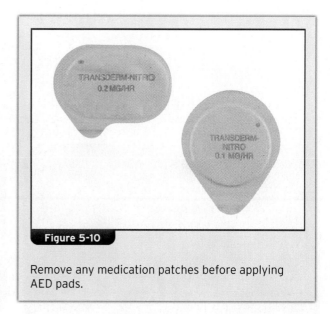

Figure 5-10

Remove any medication patches before applying AED pads.

patches may block the delivery of energy from the pads to the heart, they need to be removed and the skin wiped dry before attaching the AED pads ( ▲ Figure 5-10 ).

## Implanted Devices

Implanted pacemakers and defibrillators are small devices placed underneath the skin of people with certain

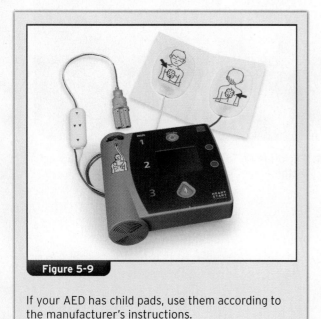

Figure 5-9

If your AED has child pads, use them according to the manufacturer's instructions.

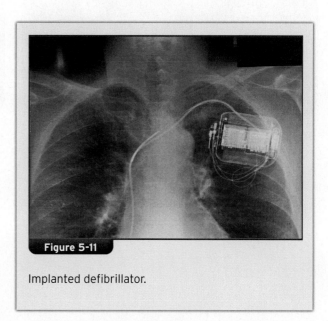

Figure 5-11

Implanted defibrillator.

types of heart disease ( ◄ Figure 5-11 ). These devices can often be seen or felt when the chest is exposed. Avoid placing the pads directly over these devices whenever possible. If an implanted defibrillator is discharging, you may see the victim twitching periodically. Allow the implanted unit to stop before using your AED.

## AED Maintenance

Periodic inspection of your AED can ensure that the device has the necessary supplies and is in proper working condition ( ►Figure 5-12 ). AEDs conduct automatic internal checks and provide visual indications that the unit is ready and functioning properly. You do not need to turn the device on daily to check it as part of any inspection. Doing so will only wear down the battery.

AED supplies should include items such as the following:

- Two sets of electrode pads with expiration dates that are not expired
- Extra battery
- Razor
- Hand towel

Other items that should be considered are a breathing device (for example, a mask or shield) and medical exam gloves.

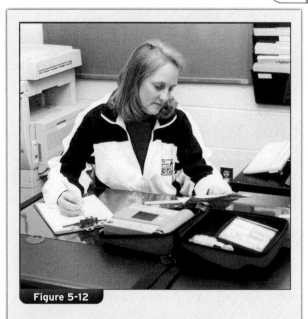

**Figure 5-12**

Inspect your AED daily to make sure it is in working condition and has the necessary supplies.

# prep kit

## ▶ Key Terms

<u>automated external defibrillator (AED)</u> Device capable of analyzing the heart rhythm and providing a shock.
<u>defibrillation</u> The electrical shock administered by an AED to reestablish a normal heart rhythm.

## ▶ Assessment in Action

A 45-year-old coworker suddenly collapses during lunch. You and several other coworkers witness this event. You check the victim and determine that he is not breathing. Your company has recently implemented an AED program, and you and other coworkers have been trained. This person needs your help to save his life.
*Directions:* Circle Yes if you agree with the statement, and circle No if you disagree.

Yes No 1. As soon as you determine that the coworker is unresponsive, you should send someone to call 9-1-1 and retrieve the AED.

Yes No 2. CPR should be performed for at least 2 minutes even if the AED is readily available.

Yes No 3. The AED pads can be applied over the top of the victim's T-shirt.

Yes No 4. If you receive a prompt from the AED that reads "Check Electrodes," the device may be indicating im-

proper placement or poor connection.

Yes No 5. This victim is not old enough to require the use of an AED.

*Answers:* 1. Yes; 2. No; 3. No; 4. Yes; 5. No

## ▶ Check Your Knowledge

*Directions:* Circle Yes if you agree with the statement, and circle No if you disagree.

Yes No 1. The earlier defibrillation occurs, the better the victim's chance of survival.

Yes No 2. An AED is only to be applied to a victim who is unresponsive and not breathing.

Yes No 3. CPR is not needed if you are sure an AED will be available in 3 to 4 minutes.

Yes No 4. AEDs require the operator to know how to interpret heart rhythms.

Yes No 5. Because all AEDs are different, the basic steps of operation are also different.

Yes No 6. The AED pads (electrodes) need to be attached to a dry chest.

Yes No 7. Two electrode pads are placed on the left side of the victim's chest.

Yes No 8. Batteries and pads have expiration dates you should be aware of.

Yes No 9. An AED can still be used if an implanted pacemaker is present.

Yes No 10. You need to turn the AED on daily as part of a routine inspection.

*Answers:* 1. Yes; 2. Yes; 3. No; 4. No; 5. No; 6. Yes; 7. No; 8. Yes; 9. Yes; 10. No

## ▶ Cardiac Arrest

### What to Look For

• Unresponsiveness
• Not breathing

### What to Do

1. Perform CPR until an AED is available.
2. Turn on the AED.
3. Apply the pads.
4. Analyze the heart rhythm.
5. Administer a shock if needed.
6. Perform CPR for five cycles (2 minutes).
7. Recheck.

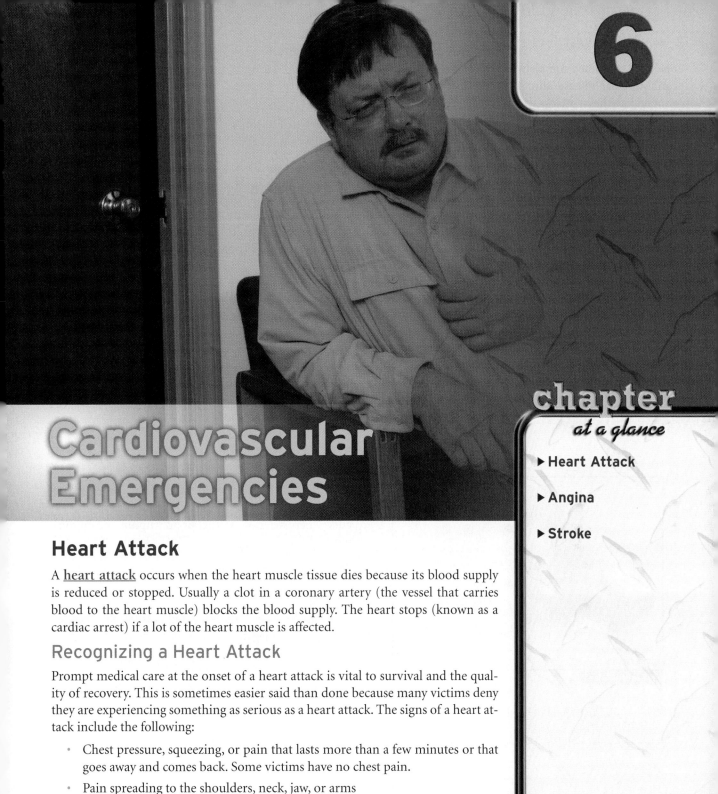

# Cardiovascular Emergencies

## Heart Attack

A <u>heart attack</u> occurs when the heart muscle tissue dies because its blood supply is reduced or stopped. Usually a clot in a coronary artery (the vessel that carries blood to the heart muscle) blocks the blood supply. The heart stops (known as a cardiac arrest) if a lot of the heart muscle is affected.

### Recognizing a Heart Attack

Prompt medical care at the onset of a heart attack is vital to survival and the quality of recovery. This is sometimes easier said than done because many victims deny they are experiencing something as serious as a heart attack. The signs of a heart attack include the following:

- Chest pressure, squeezing, or pain that lasts more than a few minutes or that goes away and comes back. Some victims have no chest pain.
- Pain spreading to the shoulders, neck, jaw, or arms
- Dizziness, sweating, nausea
- Shortness of breath

Most women do not have the classic signs of heart attack seen in men. Instead, they often have severe fatigue, upset stomach, and shortness of breath. Only about one third of women complain of severe chest pain. While cardiovascular disease affects both sexes equally, when women have heart attacks they are more likely than men to die.

## Care for a Heart Attack

To care for a heart attack victim:

1. Seek medical care by calling 9-1-1. Medications to dissolve a clot are available but must be given early.
2. Help the victim into the most comfortable resting position ( ▼ Figure 6-1 ).
3. If the victim is alert, able to swallow, and not allergic to aspirin, give one adult aspirin or two to four chewable children's aspirin.
4. If the victim has prescribed medication for heart disease, such as nitroglycerin, help the victim use it.
5. Monitor breathing.

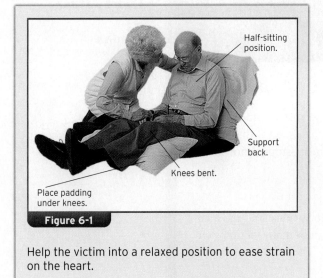

Half-sitting position.

Support back.

Knees bent.

Place padding under knees.

**Figure 6-1**

Help the victim into a relaxed position to ease strain on the heart.

## Angina

Angina is chest pain associated with heart disease that occurs when the heart muscle does not get enough blood. Angina is brought on by physical activity, exposure to cold, or emotional stress.

### Recognizing Angina

The signs of angina are similar to those of a heart attack, but the pain seldom lasts longer than 10 minutes and almost always is relieved by nitroglycerin (a prescribed medication).

### Care for Angina

To care for a victim with angina:

1. Have the victim rest.
2. If a victim has his or her own nitroglycerin, help the victim use it.
3. If the pain continues beyond 10 minutes, suspect a heart attack and call 9-1-1.

## Stroke

A stroke, also called a brain attack, occurs when part of the blood flow to the brain is suddenly cut off. This occurs when arteries in the brain rupture or become blocked ( ▶Figure 6-2 ).

### Recognizing Stroke

The signs of a stroke include the following:

- Sudden weakness or numbness of the face, an arm, or a leg on one side of the body
- Blurred or decreased vision, especially on one side of the visual field
- Problems speaking
- Dizziness or loss of balance
- Sudden, severe headache

## Sudden Illnesses

### Type of Condition Suspected?

**Heart Attack**

- Call 9-1-1.
- Help victim into a comfortable position.
- Loosen any tight clothing.
- Give one adult aspirin or two to four children's aspirin.
- Assist victim with his or her prescribed medication.
- Monitor breathing.

**Stroke**

- Call 9-1-1.
- If responsive, help victim onto his or her back with head and shoulders slightly elevated.
- If unresponsive, move victim onto his or her side.

## Care for Stroke

To care for a stroke victim:

1. Call 9-1-1.

2. If the victim is responsive, lay the victim on his or her back with the head and shoulders slightly elevated.

3. If the victim is unresponsive, open the airway, check breathing, and provide care accordingly. If the unresponsive victim is breathing, place the victim on his or her side (recovery position) to keep the airway clear.

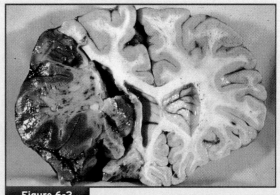

**Figure 6-2**

Severe brain hemorrhage causing a stroke.

# prep kit

## ▶ Heart Attack

### What to Look For

- Chest pressure, squeezing, or pain
- Pain spreading to shoulders, neck, jaw, or arms
- Dizziness, sweating, nausea
- Shortness of breath

### What to Do

1. Help victim take his or her prescribed medication.
2. Call 9-1-1.
3. Help victim into a comfortable position.
4. Give one adult or two to four children's aspirin.
5. Monitor breathing.

## ▶ Angina

### What to Look For

- Chest pain similar to a heart attack
- Pain seldom lasts longer than 10 minutes

### What to Do

1. Have victim rest.
2. If victim has his or her own nitroglycerin, help the victim use it.
3. If pain continues beyond 10 minutes, suspect a heart attack and call 9-1-1.

## ▶ Stroke

### What to Look For

- Sudden weakness or numbness of the face, an arm, or a leg on one side of the body
- Blurred or decreased vision
- Problems speaking
- Dizziness or loss of balance
- Sudden, severe headache

### What to Do

1. Call 9-1-1.
2. If responsive, help victim into a comfortable position with head and shoulders slightly raised.
3. If unresponsive, move onto his or her side.

## ▶ Key Terms

<u>angina</u> Chest pain caused by a lack of blood to the heart muscle.

<u>heart attack</u> Death of a part of the heart muscle.

<u>stroke</u> A blockage or rupture of arteries in the brain.

## ▶ Assessment in Action

A 50-year-old coworker is experiencing chest pain and nausea. He says that it started about an hour ago and has not let up. He believes it may just be indigestion. He describes the pain as "something pressing on my chest."

*Directions:* Circle Yes if you agree with the statement, and circle No if you disagree.

Yes No **1.** Have him lie down for 30 minutes to see if the pain subsides.

Yes No **2.** Check to see if his pupils are unequal.

Yes No **3.** His signs could indicate a heart attack.

Yes No **4.** Help the victim take an aspirin, and call EMS.

Yes No **5.** Heart attack victims often resist the idea that they need medical care.

*Answers:* **1.** No; **2.** No; **3.** Yes; **4.** Yes; **5.** Yes

## ▶ Check Your Knowledge

*Directions:* Circle Yes if you agree with the statement, and circle No if you disagree.

Yes No **1.** Heart attack victims can experience chest pain.

Yes No **2.** You can help the victim of chest pain take his or her nitroglycerin.

Yes No **3.** A responsive stroke victim should lie down with his or her head slightly raised.

Yes No **4.** Nitroglycerin may relieve chest pain associated with angina.

*Answers:* **1.** Yes; **2.** Yes; **3.** Yes; **4.** Yes

# index

Note: *f* or *t* with page number indicates figures and tables respectively.

## Chapter 1
Opener Courtesy of Larry Newell; 1-1 Used with permission from Cathy Hall; 1-2 Courtesy of Ellis and Associates.

## Chapter 2
Opener © Peter Steiner/Alamy Images.

## Chapter 3
Opener © Ingram Publishing/age fotostock.

## Chapter 4
Opener Courtesy of Larry Newell; 4-5 © Jones and Bartlett Publishers. Photographed by Kimberly Potvin.

## Chapter 5
Opener Courtesy of Larry Newell; 5-2 American Heart Association; 5-9 Courtesy of Phillips Medical Systems. All rights reserved.

# Notes

# Notes

# Notes

# Notes

# Notes

# Notes

# Notes

# Notes

# Notes

# Notes

# Notes